Celery Juicing

A Beginner's Guide and Review for Women

mf

copyright © 2020 Larry Jamesonn

All rights reserved No part of this guide may be reproduced, or stored in a retrieval system, or transmitted in any form or by any means, electronic, mechanical, photocopying, recording, or otherwise, without express written permission of the publisher.

Disclaimer

By reading this disclaimer, you are accepting the terms of the disclaimer in full. If you disagree with this disclaimer, please do not read the guide.

All of the content within this guide is provided for informational and educational purposes only, and should not be accepted as independent medical or other professional advice. The author is not a doctor, physician, nurse, mental health provider, or registered nutritionist/dietician. Therefore, using and reading this guide does not establish any form of a physician-patient relationship.

Always consult with a physician or another qualified health provider with any issues or questions you might have regarding any sort of medical condition. Do not ever disregard any qualified professional medical advice or delay seeking that advice because of anything you have read in this guide. The information in this guide is not intended to be any sort of medical advice and should not be used in lieu of any medical advice by a licensed and qualified medical professional.

The information in this guide has been compiled from a variety of known sources. However, the author cannot attest to or guarantee the accuracy of each source and thus should not be held liable for any errors or omissions.

You acknowledge that the publisher of this guide will not be held liable for any loss or damage of any kind incurred as a result of this guide or the reliance on any information provided within this guide. You acknowledge and agree that you assume all risk and responsibility for any action you undertake in response to the information in this guide.

Using this guide does not guarantee any particular result (e.g., weight loss or a cure). By reading this guide, you acknowledge that there are no guarantees to any specific outcome or results you can expect.

All product names, diet plans, or names used in this guide are for identification purposes only and are the property of their respective owners. The use of these names does not imply endorsement. All other trademarks cited herein are the property of their respective owners.

Where applicable, this guide is not intended to be a substitute for the original work of this diet plan and is, at most, a supplement to the original work for this diet plan and never a direct substitute. This guide is a personal expression of the facts of that diet plan.

Where applicable, persons shown in the cover images are stock photography models and the publisher has obtained the rights to use the images through license agreements with third-party stock image companies.

Table of Contents

Disclaimer
Table of Contents
Introduction
Chapter 1 - To Juice or Munch It
Chapter 2 – Effects on Women's Health
Chapter 3 – Celery Juicing: The Controversy
Chapter 4 – A Worthwhile Time Investment?
Chapter 5 – Extra Tips for Making Celery Juicing Work for You
Chapter 6 - Curated Recipes
Chapter 7: Choosing the Perfect Juicer for Celery Juicing
Conclusion

Introduction

Do you want to lose weight quickly, while still enjoying your favorite foods? It is possible, and you don't have to subscribe to a fad diet that you cannot sustain, either. Through celery juicing, you can prepare your body for weight loss. It can help get your bodily systems back to functioning as they should.

You may have come across the phrase "celery juicing" if you have been searching for ways to lose weight. Some controversy surrounds this practice, so you may be caught between disbelief and the desire to discover more about it. Since you have a copy of this guide, it seems that you have decided to give this a chance.

You have made the right choice. Celery juicing is a dietary practice that is a healthy and refreshing way of avoiding some of the usual calories that you take in when drinking other types of juices. You don't even have to search high and low for other ingredients to start this new health practice. If you have celery and a juicer in the kitchen, you are good to go. This guide mainly invests in assisting women in achieving their weight and health goals through drinking celery juice.

In the Celery Juicing (for Women) guide, you will discover the following topics:

- An in-depth definition of celery juicing
- The benefits of celery juicing
- How celery juicing can target women specifically
- The pros and cons of celery juicing

- An evaluation of whether the practice is worth following
- Curated recipes to keep celery juicing delightful to your taste buds
- Tips for making celery juicing work for you

So, what are you waiting for? Continue reading this quick but intensive celery juicing reading guide to take that journey towards better health. While the guide's focus is on women, anyone who is interested in the practice can read on.

Chapter 1 - To Juice or Munch It

Celery has plenty of health benefits. It does not only provide you with essential vitamins and minerals in a low-calorie package, but it also helps you battle diseases. Celery improves digestion, fights infection, and supports liver health, among many other benefits. So, it is no wonder that people have been emptying the produce section's celery to not only munch on the sticks but also to prepare celery juice. Celery juice makes it easier for you to gulp down all the nutrients early in the morning. It prepares you for the long day ahead without packing on the weight around your waist and hips.

Green Juice

While there is probably no argument here that celery is healthy, why can't we just take the sticks and munch them? Yes, it is tempting to say: Oh, I am going to drink this green thing because everyone else is doing it this way! That is not enough. This attitude is why controversies begin. When people follow a trending practice and do not know how to justify it, they surround the practice with a cloud of doubt. What if it is just a fad? Is it really worth the effort? These are valid questions that deserve answers.

Celery juice is not just a fad or trend. It has been used for centuries as a medicinal remedy in traditional medicine. In ancient Greece and Rome, celery was used to treat various ailments, including liver disease and inflammation. Even Hippocrates, the father of medicine, praised celery for its healing properties. So, it is safe to say that celery juice has been around for a long time and is backed by traditional knowledge.

Backtracking to the Source

Celery can help a lot of people improve health-wise. This is true for various health conditions. The celery may be a simple vegetable, but it has a lot of healing potential.

Celery, scientifically known as *Apium graveolens*, has a rich and fascinating history that spans continents and cultures. Belonging to the Apiaceae family, it is a marshland plant native to the Mediterranean and Middle Eastern regions. Celery has been cultivated as a vegetable since antiquity, with records indicating its use in cooking as far back as 9th century BC, in Homer's *Iliad*.

In ancient times, celery was valued more for its medicinal properties than its culinary use. Egyptians and Greeks used it as a powerful healing agent. It was also linked to death and the afterlife. Wreaths of celery leaves were found in the tomb of Tutankhamun, and Greeks used it to adorn winners of the Nemean Games, believed to be funeral games in honor of the dead.

Its journey to the North of Europe, particularly Britain, happened much later, around the 16th century, but it was only in the 19th century that celery was utilized as a principal ingredient in cuisine. The form of celery often used in modern cooking, known as Pascal celery, was developed in the 17th century.

The raw vegetable form is also potent in its own way. It has fiber that you need for proper digestion. However, when it is blended to create juice, the fiber is removed. The removal of the celery makes the celery a lot more effective in terms of health recovery after illness and other benefits. You may prefer giving your celery juice a little twist: add a little bit of the fiber in the same way that some fruit juices have a little bit of pulp. You can also add other beneficial ingredients such as ginger or lemon to enhance the flavor and health benefits of your green juice.

Advantages of Drinking Celery Juice

When you drink celery juice, you are more likely to absorb more content than when you eat the stalks. When taking in the solid form, you may easily get fed up after a little bit of chewing. Even when you still feel like eating celery, you may find yourself full before you have ingested enough nutrients. In juice form, you can take in more nutrients at any given time.

Unlike other drinks, celery juice is not harsh on your stomach. You can even drink it on an empty stomach. It is at its most powerful when you drink it without mixing it with other ingredients. However, you may flavor it with other vegetable juices, such as those extracted from cilantro, kale, parsley, spinach, and more. Sometimes, people also mix it with fruits, such as apples. Some of the recipes included in this guide have taken advantage of the tangy taste of apples to keep the celery juice taste fresh without packing in calories.

Celery juice also increases your bile content. This increase is necessary for breaking down fats and eliminating waste. So, you could say that celery juicing promotes liver health. It also comes with antioxidant and anti-inflammatory properties, which are useful in keeping you healthy and illness-free. Sometimes, you need to get these benefits from supplements, but here they are in a purely natural form.

Bile is also good for removing toxins from the body. When you drink celery juice, it helps remove various impurities from your bloodstream and the rest of your body. This process can help clear up your skin and rid it of acne breakouts or other blemishes. What's more, celery juice also contains vitamins A, C, and K, which are all beneficial for maintaining healthy skin. So, by drinking celery juice regularly, you can achieve clear and glowing skin.

Moreover, celery juice is packed with essential minerals like potassium, magnesium, and calcium. These minerals are necessary for maintaining healthy bones and muscles.

Potassium, magnesium, and calcium are essential minerals that play a critical role in overall health and well-being.

Potassium plays a vital role in maintaining fluid balance, nerve signals, and muscle contractions in the body. It helps to maintain a healthy blood pressure by counteracting the effects of sodium and reducing the risks associated with heart disease. Furthermore, it supports heart health by helping the heart to pump blood. Evidence suggests that a potassium-rich diet can help prevent stroke and osteoporosis and mitigate the effects of kidney stones.

Magnesium is involved in more than 300 enzymatic reactions in the body, including protein synthesis, muscle and nerve function, blood glucose control, and blood pressure regulation. It aids in the production of energy and plays a significant role in the structural development of bones. Consuming an adequate amount of magnesium can help prevent chronic diseases such as Alzheimer's disease, type 2 diabetes, cardiovascular disease, and migraine.

Calcium is the most abundant mineral in the body. It is vital for building and maintaining strong bones and teeth, as 99% of the body's calcium is stored in the bones and teeth. Furthermore, it plays a role in maintaining healthy communication between the brain and other parts of the body. It helps blood vessels move blood throughout the body and aids in releasing hormones and enzymes that affect almost every function in the human body. Calcium also plays a role in muscle function and supports nerve signaling.

These minerals are naturally present in celery juice, making it a healthful addition to your diet. Including celery juice in your dietary regimen ensures you're getting these essential minerals in their natural form, which is more bioavailable, meaning the body can absorb and utilize them more effectively. Consuming them in a natural form, as opposed to supplements, may also reduce the risk of overconsumption, which can lead to health issues. Therefore, drinking celery juice is not only refreshing but also a convenient way to enhance your daily mineral intake and bolster your overall health.

By incorporating celery juice into your diet, you can help prevent conditions like osteoporosis and arthritis. Additionally, celery juice contains high levels of vitamin C, which boosts the immune system and helps fight off infections and diseases.

Chapter 2 – Effects on Women's Health

Celery juicing is beneficial to everyone. However, we are going to zero in just a tad more on women in this guide.

How does celery juicing affect the health of women?

Celery juicing is not necessarily simply targeted at women. It is recommended to any person who is interested in celery's anti-inflammatory properties. However, this guide will show you that we recognize just how more women are seeking weight-loss and health boost strategies.

Why is this the case?

Well, women have been more affected by the fluctuations of hormones than men. They have to go through menstruation, pregnancies, menopause, and many other special events that skew their hormonal balance. You should also think about those who have conditions that create an imbalance at any given point in time, such as polycystic ovary syndrome.

When a woman is going through a hormonal imbalance, they are likely to feel surges in their appetite. They will crave sweets and salty foods that will wreak havoc on their bodies.

Cravings in women, particularly for sweet or salty foods, can be attributed to a multitude of factors. The most common of these is hormonal fluctuations, as mentioned above, which occur as women go through different stages of their menstrual cycle, pregnancy, and menopause.

Hormones such as estrogen and progesterone ebb and flow throughout the menstrual cycle, influencing various bodily functions including mood, appetite, and even taste preferences. During the luteal phase (the week or so before menstruation), progesterone levels peak, causing an increase in appetite and a predilection for high-fat, high-sugar foods. This is the body's way of preparing for potential pregnancy by storing energy.

Similar hormonal shifts occur during pregnancy. For instance, increasing levels of human chorionic gonadotropin (hCG) in the early stages of pregnancy are believed to be responsible for food cravings. Additionally, pregnancy is a time of heightened sense of taste and smell, which can steer food preferences.

Lastly, during menopause, as estrogen levels decline, women may experience changes in taste and an increased desire for savory foods.

Beyond hormones, cravings can be influenced by nutritional deficiencies. For example, a craving for chocolate could indicate a deficiency in magnesium, while a longing for red meat might signify low iron levels.

It's also worth noting that cravings can be linked to emotional states. Stress, boredom, and emotional distress can all trigger cravings as eating certain foods releases feel-good hormones like serotonin, leading to temporary emotional relief.

Understanding the root cause of cravings can help women navigate them more effectively, making healthier choices that align with their overall wellness goals. While it's okay to indulge cravings in moderation, consistently consuming high-fat, high-sugar foods can lead to weight gain and other health concerns. Therefore, it's crucial to balance cravings with a nutritious diet, including plenty of fruits, vegetables, whole grains, and lean proteins.

Too much sugar and salt in the body contribute to serious conditions, such as diabetes and hypertension. Yes, men can also develop these conditions when they do not have healthy eating habits, but they do not experience the hormonal fluctuations that women go through.

Hormonal imbalance in women can manifest in various ways and is often deeply connected to their overall health and well-being. This imbalance can be the result of natural processes, such as menstruation, pregnancy, and menopause, or it can be due to certain conditions like polycystic ovary syndrome (PCOS). Hormonal fluctuations can lead to a range of symptoms including mood swings, fatigue, skin problems, weight gain, and irregular periods. As such, a nutritional approach to balancing hormones can be highly beneficial. Incorporating foods like celery, known for its anti-inflammatory properties, can help regulate hormonal imbalances and alleviate some of the associated symptoms. The natural sodium in celery can also help curb cravings for salty foods, thus promoting a healthier diet. It's important to note that each individual's response to food can differ, so it's always recommended to consult with a healthcare provider or a registered dietitian when making significant dietary changes.

Why else do women feel they have to find an easily sustainable diet?

It also has something to do with the acceptable, albeit stereotypical, roles that women play in society. They are mothers and caregivers. Though men may be great providers, the stress of actually making a house run a certain way is often left on the shoulders of women. I am not saying that this is what each household has in effect, but even in the most equal-rights and equal-role family, the woman's body is the one geared to wake up to a baby's cry, for example.

Because of these roles, you will find women less able to free themselves to go to the gym when kids at home are waiting for them. Some do make this work, but often some just stay in with the kids to save money twice: one, for not paying for a gym membership, and two, for not hiring a nanny to care for the kids.

So, women need something easy to commit to that they can incorporate into their busy role-juggling timetable.

Celery juicing is a practical and sustainable option because:

- Certainly, gulping down a glass of celery juice is quick and healthy. A woman can go back to her multiple duties right away.
- It makes her feel fuller so that she does not end up binging or stress eating.
- It prevents hypertension and lowers bad cholesterol.

- Daily replacing that milkshake with celery juice can start showing its results through weight loss. Yes, it can be slow, but sure.
- It refreshes you and provides a little flavor to what otherwise will be plain water for you.
- It lowers your probability of developing diabetes and heart disease.

So, in the morning, before you take that run, you may want to take a glass of celery juice. Add a low-calorie solid food to put some food in your stomach if you are not used to a completely liquid diet. On the other hand, you may stick to the glass of celery juice alone if you are used to eating a little at a time.

To make it official:

Celery juice is excellent for you because it helps regularize bodily functions. This very description, it can be helpful to women who have some hormonal imbalances. Being able to relax at the possibility of having a sustainable diet control strategy can also ease the stress a bit. Women have to lose some weight and be more relaxed to reduce the symptoms of polycystic ovaries and other hormonal imbalances.

Chapter 3 – Celery Juicing: The Controversy

Not everyone is sold out on celery juicing, and we need to face that controversy head-on. Here are the pros and cons of celery juice.

Let us begin with the pros.

One: The most common selling point of celery juicing is that it can help you lose weight. Juicing, as a whole, provides you with a means of absorbing more nutrients from celery without you getting fed up as you may quickly do so with the solid form. Celery also has fewer calories than other juices, which may include sugary fruits such as mango.

Two: Celery juice helps you digest food more quickly because it increases stomach acid. Those with high protein diets will more likely benefit because stomach acid is necessary for breaking down protein. Just because there is an acid increase does not mean you will be experiencing acid reflux or ulcers. On the contrary, you will be getting more gastric mucus that will protect or heal you from such conditions.

Three: Celery juice has anti-inflammatory properties. It can get rid of the conditions that have inflammation as their primary symptom. So, it can help you recover from gout, arthritis, and the like.

Four: Full of potent antioxidants, celery juice, has been reported to have cancer-fighting properties. Apigenin, a flavonoid found in celery, is said to be capable of killing cancer cells. Its alkalizing content further helps it prevent chronic diseases.

Five: Because celery helps reduce fat buildup in the liver, it helps boost the organ's health.

Six: It helps battle infections of all kinds, including reproductive, digestive, and urinary infections. It does this by fighting microbes and reducing uric acid.

Seventh: It lowers cholesterol and blood pressure, thus contributing to your cardiovascular health. The 3-n-butylphthalide (BuPh) compound in celery reduces bad cholesterol (LDL). Celery also contains a muscle relaxant that aids the blood vessels in quickly expanding and contracting.

Eighth: It helps in clearing some skin problems, including eczema and acne. This property is especially helpful to women who have been struggling with hormonal imbalances.

Ninth: It boosts relaxation that can help soothe your nerves, allowing you to sleep better. Women are more likely to experience sleeping problems. Celery juice, added to a healthy sleep ritual, can help reduce instances of insomnia the natural way.

Tenth: Celery juice detoxifies your body in many ways. An active component of celery, Molybdenum, makes this possible. The same celery component helps in repairing teeth minerals to preserve teeth.

What are the benefits that specifically target women?

All of the seven main points that support the value of drinking celery juice apply to any person, regardless of age and gender. However, women can gain some extra benefits from drinking celery juice.

- Most studies reveal that celery juice has fertility benefits for women. While it may not solely solve your fertility problems, adding it to your daily diet can help revert your bodily functions to normal. Such a function includes a boost in your fertility.
- Celery juice helps in reducing bloating for women during menstruation. The presence of phthalides and phytonutrients in celery can help regulate hormones and alleviate inflammation associated with bloating. This property makes celery a good choice for women who experience discomfort
- It is an easy solution to working moms who have to juggle their careers, their children, and their partners. Celery juice can undoubtedly benefit the 21st-century woman.
- Some women can attest that the celery juicing practice has reduced the cramps they usually feel before a period. They were not able to explain why exactly, but the effects have manifested after at least two or three months of drinking celery juice daily.

Even those who debunk celery juicing as an unestablished miracle worker also believe in the health properties presented by the vegetable.

But what exactly are the cons of celery juicing?

Nothing is perfect, unfortunately. Celery juicing also has some disadvantages that will prevent you from guzzling the green juice all day long.

- It has sodium content. Too much celery juice can raise your sodium levels. So, whatever benefit you have been striving for will be all for naught. You certainly will not lower your blood pressure with high sodium content.
- It gets rid of most of the fiber. Often, it just does away with it altogether. The fiber is the component that can help you the most with your digestion. It also leaves you fuller for longer. You may want a recipe that adds just a little bit of fiber, just as some fruit juices contain some pulp.
- Celery, on its own, can make for a healthy but bitter-tasting juice. So, it is better combined with other flavors, such as apple. You may not find yourself wanting to have a few glasses of celery juice, unlike other fruit juices. Therefore, this may limit how much you can enjoy the health benefits of celery juice.
- Celery juicing also has its drawbacks in terms of sustainability. As much as it is healthy for your body, growing celery can be resource-intensive and requires a lot of water.
- A high concentration of celery juice can raise sugar levels because concentrated celery contains a lot more sugar than it naturally has as a solid. Celery juicing has been attempting to get as many nutrients into one glass. However, it also concentrates the sugar level while lowering the fiber.

- Psoralen in celery can cause oversensitivity to UV rays when you have drunk too much celery juice. Overexposure to UV rays can lead to skin irritation, rashes, and even sunburns.
- In some individuals, celery juice can cause bloating or digestive discomfort.

Despite these potential cons, many people still swear by the benefits of celery juicing and have incorporated it into their daily routines.

Calling a truce

Of course, celery juice is more than just a fad. It contains nutrients in one delicious glass of refreshing juice. Make some adjustments to your recipe to increase the benefits and lower the negative issues that are associated with this new healthy trend.

- Handpick fresh celery yourself. You want to know where your ingredient is coming from.
- Wash your celery thoroughly before you put it in the blender.
- Do not get rid of all the fiber. You need it to be full fast, which can, in turn, aid in weight loss.
- Pack in the nutrients without leaving the juice as too concentrated. Add just a little bit more water or some ice cubes.
- Mix it up with a low-calorie fruit for better taste. For the low calorie ideal, mix the celery with ginger, lemon, or cucumber.

- Take out the foam that forms on top of the juice, because it has been reported to taste terrible. While you want to be healthy as quickly as possible, you don't want to give up so early in the game.
- When mixing with another fruit, alternate between that fruit and celery. Yes, you will be blending the fruit and celery anyway. However, this is found useful by some who have tried it.
- Drink your celery juice within 24 hours of blending it. Do not let it stay for longer than that.
- Drink it as a breakfast picker-upper.
- Sip it slowly in 30 minutes, instead of guzzling it down. It does have a certain aftertaste, which may take a while to get used to – especially for those who have not eaten celery before.

Then, you leave it like that. Do not drink any more of the celery juice for the day. 16 oz. glass should be enough for the day.

Record your reactions, chosen recipes, and effects (immediate or otherwise). Documentation may be the only way to finally prove that while celery juice is not a miracle juice like some people claim it is, it is genuinely capable of delivering all the pros that have been listed in this chapter.

Chapter 4 – A Worthwhile Time Investment?

Now that we know the pros and cons of celery juicing, we pause to ask: is it worthwhile to prepare the drink every morning?

It is a time investment because instead of guzzling through a glass of milk or your cup of Instant Coffee before you go to work, you have to go through the process of celery juicing.

The steps go like this:

- Wash the celery thoroughly
- Cut into small cubes
- Put into your slow-masticating juicer
- Blend alone or with other vegetables
- Consider adding fruits alternately
- Add ice cubes as desired
- Remove the foam on top
- Pour into a glass
- Drink

Compare that to just pouring fresh milk into a glass or pouring hot water onto your coffee granules. It is a time investment. Some of you will go through it once a day only, but some may opt to drink celery juice twice a day. This ritual has to be repeated the following day because celery juice cannot be kept for more than 24 hours.

So, let us cut to the chase. It is worth it.

Even those who have been following a vegan diet recognize that, yes, they are healthy, but adding celery juice to their diet still adds extra oomph. Those who have started a celery diet on top of their already healthy lifestyle have noticed additional benefits.

But what is stopping some people from starting a celery juice habit?

- Many of the experiences are undocumented. So, people are still relying on old studies regarding the use of liquified celery.
- The taste can put people off when they attempt to start the habit.
- It can mean buying a slow-masticating juicer, which is expensive. So, not only is it a time investment, but it also costs some money. Celery prices have also risen because of the trend.
- It takes a lot of time to prepare in the mornings before work.

The points above, however, can be given solutions.

- More people are now posting their personal experiences with celery juice. Some are positive, and some are negative. So, focus on the details of their experiences. Some posters explain why the experience has benefitted them.
- The taste can be off putting, but you are allowed to add fruits and other vegetables. You may also make the drink a little less concentrated. Moreover, the taste becomes more manageable when you remove the foam from the top.
- While some slow masticating juicers often cost hundreds of dollars, some going for more than 600

USD, you can find affordable ones at less than 100 USD. You may want to start with a starter juicer before you can commit.
- It is still best to drink your celery juice straight from the juicer. However, if this is not possible, you still have until 24 hours to finish the juice. Refrigerate the juice overnight. In the morning, you may drink it right away or add a garnish or flavor if you prefer so.

Celery juicing may present fundamental issues to some, but it is a good time and money investment.

Chapter 5 – Extra Tips for Making Celery Juicing Work for You

As we wind down a little towards the actual celery juice recipes, here are some a few tips to guide you along:

- Slow masticating juicers are best in maximizing the nutrients you get from your celery. Centrifugal juicers, on the other hand, will expose your celery to heat and oxygen. Using them is not advisable because it may further shorten the already brief shelf life of your celery juice.
- Do not drink the celery juice if it starts tasting vinegary. You need only to take small sips at a time, anyway. A bubbly, carbonated look also means you should not dare drink it anymore.
- You can make your celery juice last up to two to three days if you store it in a tightly lidded Mason jar. Otherwise, you should take it within 24 hours.
- While you may drink your glass of celery juice at any time during the day, the best time to take it is in the morning at 15 minutes before eating breakfast.
- At the moment, you cannot get hold of pure celery juice in stores. You have to make your own. However, you may start seeing celery juice mixed with something else. The top option is to make your celery juice.
- It is best to pair up your celery juice habit with an overall healthy lifestyle. This means exercise regularly, sleep well, and eat a balanced, low-calorie diet.

As more studies on celery juice get conducted, more tips should start popping up. The curated recipes in the next chapter will help you get started.

Chapter 6 - Curated Recipes

Celery Ginger Juice

Ingredients

- 1 small bunch celery (or 1 heart)
- 1/2 English cucumber
- 1 large green apple
- 1/2 lemon
- 1 -inch knob of ginger

Instructions

- If your juicer has a "high" and "low" setting, run the celery and cucumber through first on the LOW setting.
- Then switch it to HIGH and run the apple, lemon, and ginger through the juicer. I like to sandwich the piece of ginger between the apple and lemon so that it stays put and is easier to juice.
- Drink the juice right away, or save it in an airtight mason jar for up to 24 hours in the fridge.

Apply and Celery Juice with Ginger

Ingredients

- 2 celery ribs, cut into approximately 2-inches
- 1 apple, halved and cored into large pieces
- 1 slice of ginger
- 1/2 bunch of parsley
- 1 tablespoon lemon juice

Instructions

- Juice all the ingredients in a juicer
- Stir in the lemon juice.

Celery Apple Kale Lemon

Ingredients

- 3 medium-sized apples
- 1 cup of chopped celery
- 1 cup of kale
- 1/2 medium-sized lemon

Instructions

- In an electric juicer, juice the celery with the ingredients
- Add the lemon

Blood Care Juice

Ingredients:

- 1 cup of chopped celery
- 1 kiwi
- 1/2 cup of kale
- 1/2 cup of angelica
- 1 or 2 medium-sized apples

Instructions

- In an electric juicer, juice the celery with the ingredients

Popeye Celery Juice Recipe

Ingredients:

- 1 cup of chopped celery
- 1 cup of spinach
- 3 Medium-sized apples

Instructions

- In an electric juicer, juice the celery with the ingredients

Celery Pineapple Mint Juice

Ingredients:

- 3 celery stalks
- 1 cup of pineapple chunks
- A handful of fresh mint

Instructions:

- Juice the celery stalks, pineapple chunks, and mint using an electric juicer.

Celery Beetroot Carrot Juice

Ingredients:

- 2 celery stalks
- 1 small beetroot
- 2 medium-sized carrots

Instructions:

- Put the celery, beetroot, and carrots in an electric juicer and extract the juice.

Celery Pear Ginger Juice

Ingredients:

- 3 celery stalks
- 2 ripe pears
- 1 inch of fresh ginger

Instructions:

- Juice the celery stalks, pears, and ginger using an electric juicer.

Celery Cucumber Lemon Detox Juice

Ingredients:

- 4 celery stalks
- 1 cucumber
- Juice of 1 lemon

Instructions:

- Put the celery and cucumber in an electric juicer and extract the juice. Stir in the lemon juice.

Celery Blueberry Antioxidant Juice

Ingredients:

- 3 celery stalks
- 1 cup of blueberries

Instructions:

- Put the celery stalks and blueberries in an electric juicer and extract the juice.

Celery Grapefruit Vitamin Boost Juice

Ingredients:

- 4 celery stalks
- 1 large grapefruit

Instructions:

- Peel the grapefruit and put it in an electric juicer with the celery stalks. Extract the juice.

Celery Apple Cleanse Juice

Ingredients:

- 4 celery stalks
- 2 large apples

Instructions:

- Cut the apples into large pieces and juice them with the celery stalks using an electric juicer.

Celery Carrot Immunity Juice

Ingredients:

- 3 celery stalks
- 2 large carrots

Instructions:

- Juice the celery stalks and carrots using an electric juicer.

Celery Mango Tropical Juice

Ingredients:

- 3 celery stalks
- 1 cup of mango chunks

Instructions:

- Put the celery stalks and mango chunks in an electric juicer and extract the juice.

Celery Pomegranate Antioxidant Juice

Ingredients:

- 4 celery stalks
- 1 cup of pomegranate seeds

Instructions:

- Put the celery stalks and pomegranate seeds in an electric juicer and extract the juice.

Chapter 7 - Choosing the Perfect Juicer for Celery Juicing

When it comes to juicing celery, not just any juicer will do. There are certain factors to consider to ensure that you're getting the most out of your celery juice and your juicer. Here are some tips to help you choose the perfect juicer for celery juicing.

1. Masticating vs. Centrifugal Juicers

There are two main types of juicers: masticating and centrifugal. Masticating juicers, also known as slow or cold-press juicers, use a slow, crushing and squeezing method to extract juice, which can preserve more nutrients and enzymes. They are ideal for juicing leafy greens like celery as they extract maximum juice and retain more nutrients. In contrast, centrifugal juicers use a fast spinning blade which can generate heat, thereby potentially losing nutrients.

2. Yield and Pulp Ejection

Consider a juicer that offers high juice yield, as the goal is to extract the maximum amount of juice from the celery. Also, models with external pulp ejection systems allow for continuous juicing as you don't have to stop to empty out the pulp.

3. Noise Level

Juicers can be quite noisy, especially centrifugal models. If noise is a concern for you, consider a slow/masticating juicer, which tends to operate more quietly.

4. Size and Storage

The size of the juicer may factor into your decision, depending on your kitchen space. Some juicers are bulky and take up a lot of counter space, while others are more compact. Also, consider how easy it is to assemble and disassemble for storage.

5. Ease of Cleaning

Juicing should be a joy and not a chore. Thus, opt for a juicer that is easy to clean, with removable parts that are dishwasher-safe, to make the cleanup process easier.

6. Price

Lastly, the price can be a determining factor. While high-end juicers often offer more features and yield more juice, there are also budget-friendly options available that do a decent job.

7. Warranty

A long warranty period is a good indication of the manufacturer's confidence in the product. It's a safety net that can save you money on repairs or replacement if the juicer breaks down.

Before making a purchase, it's advisable to read customer reviews and do some research to understand the pros and cons of different models. You can also visit a store to see the juicers in action, or even try juicing some celery. Remember, the best juicer for you is one that suits your specific needs and preferences.

Conclusion

Juicing is a great way to incorporate more fruits and vegetables into your diet. Celery, in particular, is a versatile ingredient that can be added to many juice recipes for its numerous health benefits. From aiding digestion and detoxifying the body to boosting immunity and providing essential vitamins and antioxidants, celery should definitely be a staple in any juicing regimen.

Experiment with different combinations of fruits and vegetables to find your favorite celery juice recipe. And remember, using an electric juicer is the best way to get the most nutrients out of your produce. So go ahead and give these celery juice recipes a try for a delicious and nutritious addition to your daily routine! So let's enjoy juicing!! Happy Juicing !!

Printed in Great Britain
by Amazon